HOW TO BECOME A SUPERB DOCTOR

A MUST READ BOOK FOR MEDICAL STUDENTS AND DOCTORS

KAMRAN KHAN

Clever Fox®
PUBLISHING

Chennai • Bangalore

CLEVER FOX PUBLISHING
Chennai, India

Published by CLEVER FOX PUBLISHING 2025

ISBN: 978-93-6707-263-9

To my parents,
for always loving and supporting me.

FOREWORD

In my long journey as a cardiologist, spanning over five decades, I have seen medicine evolve from simple diagnostics to advanced technologies. Yet, one truth remains unchanged: the heart of healing lies not just in science, but in the human touch. It is this very essence that Dr. Kamran Khan captures so beautifully in his book, "How to Become a Superb Doctor - A Must Read Book for Medical Student and Doctors."

Dr. Khan, with his many years of dedicated service in the AYUSH Department, brings a fresh and practical perspective. Drawing from real-life experiences, he reminds us that being a good doctor goes far beyond textbooks and prescriptions. The book is divided into three thoughtful sections: understanding patient expectations, building key qualities like compassion and communication, and paying attention to the little things that build trust—such as a clean clinic or a kind word at the reception.

I particularly appreciate how Dr. Khan stresses empathy and attentiveness. In cardiology, where patients often face life-altering fears, a simple act of listening can ease more pain than any pill. He warns against the pitfalls of commercial influences and urges doctors to stay true to ethical practice. These insights are timely, especially in India's growing healthcare landscape, where patient-centered care is key to building lasting relationships.

This book is a must-read for medical students, interns, and seasoned professionals alike. It serves as a gentle reminder that true excellence in medicine comes from blending knowledge with kindness. Dr. Khan's work inspires us to not only treat diseases but to nurture lives. I am honored to introduce this valuable guide and wish it reaches every aspiring healer's hands.

Dr. M. Khalilullah
Padma Shri, Padma Bhushan
Former Hon. Physician to the President of India
Chief Cardiologist, The Heart Centre
New Delhi

PREFACE

Medicine is not merely a science. It is also a deeply human art. Over the course of nearly 25 years of clinical practice, I have encountered thousands of patients. Many of them sought my care not as a first option. But as an alternative, after feeling let down by others. This recurring experience prompted a critical question: Why do patients lose faith in their doctors?

Driven by this question, I began to explore the factors behind patient dissatisfaction. I listened to patients and observed patterns. Plus, I reviewed research on doctor-patient relationships. What I discovered was both concerning and enlightening. A significant number of doctors are unaware of what patients truly expect from them. This expectation is not in terms of treatment outcomes alone. But it is also in terms of communication, empathy, integrity, and presence.

This book is born out of that realization. It is a call to action (CTA) for medical students, interns, and residents. It is also a CTA for practicing physicians to not only strive for clinical excellence, but to cultivate the human qualities that define a good doctor. Through personal experience, case observations, and thoughtful reflection, I have compiled insights. Based on these insights, I will guide young medical professionals to make a strong doctor-patient' relationship.

This work also speaks to medical educators: the values we teach matter just as much as the techniques. We place empathy, ethics, and patient-centered care at the heart of medical training. Doing this, we can shape a future generation of doctors who heal not just the body, but the whole person.

Let this book be not just a guide. But a companion on your journey to becoming not just a doctor, but a superb doctor.

Kamran Khan

ACKNOWLEDGEMENT

THE HEART BEHIND THIS WORK

There may be just one name listed as the author of the book, but it would never have been possible without the support, encouragement, and inspiration of many special people.

ARISHA AND ZAINAB, my lovely daughters. In you, I see the finest part of me. You are my life's most beautiful gift. Everything I do is for you, and your love fuels every word I write.

YASHFEEN FATIMA, my dear niece. Thank you for being a constant source of joy and motivation in my life.

EVERYONE AT CLEVERFOX PUBLISHING- Thank you for your consistent support, professionalism, and belief in this project. Your encouragement meant a lot.

SHWETA DEY, thank you for standing by this book and by me. Your clarity and support helped shape the final version in ways I deeply appreciate.

GITANJALI GUPTA, your insight, vision, and guidance have influenced this book in more ways than I can count. Thank you for giving words to my thoughts and gently shaping my emotions into expression. You helped me turn thoughts into language and silence into meaning.

MOHD. RASHID and NITESH SHARMA, my friends and pillars of support. Thank you for always being there and offering your valuable help whenever needed.

Dr. RAVI KHANNA (Paediatrician and Neonatologist)—I had the honour of working with you early in my career. This book may reflect my thoughts, but its heart is inspired by you. Everything I have described here—organization, innovation, adaptability, early adoption of technology, and above all, integrity—you have consistently lived by. As I completed the final draft, I realised this book mirrors the values you embody.

READERS, thank you for taking the time to explore these pages. Your curiosity and passion are what keep medicine alive and evolving.

SHABNAM, my wife—you are good, all the way to your soul. Your patience, kindness, and deep understanding make me feel lucky every single day. Thank you for everything.

To all the **UNSEEN HANDS and SILENT SUPPORTERS**—those who offered a kind word, a moment of encouragement, or simply believed in me when I needed it most—thank you. Your presence, whether near or far, created a quiet strength that carried me through. Every message, gesture, and act of kindness became part of this journey. You may not be named here, but your contribution lives on every page of this book.

This book is a tribute to all of you. This book exists because of you!

CONTENTS

SECTION 1

PATIENT EXPECTATIONS

CHAPTER 1

CARING WITH HEART – THE ROLE OF COMPASSION IN MEDICINE

> The good physician treats the disease; the great physician treats the patient who has the disease.

In the world of medicine, knowledge is important. But it is not enough. As doctors, we focus on clinical accuracy and fast decision-making. Yet, what truly touches a patient's heart is not just our expertise, but our compassion.

A simple "I understand," or "I'm sorry to hear that," can go a long way. When we say, "This must be a lot to handle," or "How can I best support you?" we give something beyond treatment — we offer comfort. In just a few seconds, empathy builds trust and soothes anxiety. It opens doors to honest conversations.

Compassion lets us see the human behind the symptoms. It reminds our patients that they are not alone. These moments of connection — small, heartfelt, sincere — are what many remember long after the diagnosis and medication. Compassion becomes the bridge between medical care and emotional support.

Empathy, on the other hand, lets us walk briefly in our patient's shoes. It sharpens our ability to listen, to understand unspoken fears, and to ask gently, "What concerns you the most?" Asking about daily routines or meals helps make our care more personal and more powerful.

In our busy schedules, it's easy to forget what it feels like to sit on the other side of the table — to be the patient. But if we remember to connect, if we practise compassion daily, we do not only heal — we also uplift. And in doing so, we become not just good doctors, but great ones.

The best doctors are those who keep their hearts open, who take a moment to listen, and who never forget what it's like to be on the other side. Compassion is not extra work — it's the most human part of healing.

CHAPTER 2

ATTENTIVENESS – THE ART OF TRULY LISTENING

> The most basic of all human needs is the need to understand and be understood.
>
> – **Ralph G. Nichols**

A patient doesn't just want to be heard. They want to be understood. In the clinical world, we focus so much on diagnosis that we forget the importance of listening deeply. Attentiveness is an active expression of care. It means being fully present, not just hearing but truly listening. It means more than just hearing words—it means making the patients feel respected, safe, and truly seen.

When a patient speaks, they are not delivering a monologue. They hope for a conversation. They observe everything—your eye contact, your body language, the way you respond. If you look at the clock, interrupt, or appear mentally elsewhere, they know it. This is where their trust begins to fade.

Attentiveness means being present. It means listening without jumping to conclusions, and asking thoughtful follow-up questions—not just to clarify the symptoms, but to show that you care. Even when the patient drifts into unrelated matters, their words might carry hidden stressors, emotional burdens, or overlooked signs.

Never let them walk out of your chamber feeling they attended a lecture. Let them feel it was a dialogue. Let them feel that— their pain, their story, their health mattered to you—not just their lab results.

Sometimes, the greatest impact you make is not in the treatment plan you prescribe, but in the attention you give. A doctor who listens well is remembered with gratitude and respect, because healing begins with connection.

Be attentive not only for the diagnosis but for the human being in front of you. That is where the real medicine lies.

CHAPTER 3

THE HEALING POWER OF RESPECT

> Respect is how to treat everyone, not just those you want to impress.
>
> **– Richard Branson**

Respect is not just a virtue—it's the heartbeat of the doctor-patient relationship. As doctors, we often seek to heal with medicines, but kindness and respect can be just as powerful. Patients come to us with more than symptoms—they come with emotions, fears, and hopes. When we show them true respect, we do more than treat—we connect.

Respect means listening without interrupting, explaining without judging, and valuing each person's right to choose what's best for their own body. It's not about controlling the decision; it's about supporting the person making it.

When patients feel respected, they not only trust us more but also respond better to treatment and report higher satisfaction. Respect builds a bridge between medical knowledge and human care.

As doctors, we hold great power. Let's use it not only to cure, but to comfort. Respect isn't an added extra—it's a clinical tool. And like any tool, it must be used wisely, every day, with every patient.

In every consultation, let respect be the first step because healing begins with how we treat, not just what we treat.

CHAPTER 4

THE GIFT OF TIME: A PRESCRIPTION FOR PATIENT TRUST

> Time is generally the best doctor.
>
> – **Ovid**

As doctors, we find ourselves managing multiple concerns within a limited timeframe. But it is essential to accept that some patients simply require more time than others. Each patient comes with a unique set of symptoms, emotions, and questions. Instead of rushing through five tasks in ten minutes, we must pause, listen, and engage.

A patient's time is as valuable as ours. When they walk into our clinic, they expect not just a diagnosis but also the space to express their concerns. Allowing them the opportunity to ask questions and be heard during the consultation builds trust. This improves outcomes.

Short appointments may lead to miscommunication, missed diagnoses, or dissatisfaction. If patients feel unheard or hurried, their confidence in the treatment plan may diminish. On the other hand, a few extra minutes of genuine attention can make a lasting impact.

Let us reframe our approach—not just treating illnesses, but treating individuals with the respect and time they deserve. Quality care begins with quality time. The best medicine a doctor can offer is undivided attention.

CHAPTER 5

THE QUIET STRENGTH OF COURTEOUSNESS- WHERE KINDNESS MEETS CLINICAL CARE

> Too often, we underestimate the power of a touch, a smile, a kind word, a listening ear, an honest compliment, or the smallest act of caring, all of which have the potential to turn a life around.
>
> **– Leo Buscaglia,**
>
> **American author and motivational speaker**

In the world of medicine, we measure success in diagnoses, procedures, and outcomes. But what many of us forget is that behind every file lies a person—an anxious mother, a confused elderly man, a worried teenager—each carrying their own story. Courteousness, though simple and often overlooked, is one of the most powerful tools in a doctor's practice.

Patients don't just look for knowledge or efficiency. Studies consistently rank courteousness—politeness, good manners, and consideration—among the top five qualities they expect from their doctor. A warm smile, a gentle handshake, a respectful "please, have a seat," and attentive eye contact may seem like small gestures, but they can bring immense comfort.

True courtesy lives in the details. Sitting at eye level with a patient rather than towering over them. Offering water to a parched throat. Not checking the phone in the middle of a conversation. Offering a blanket when they feel cold. These are not grand acts, but they leave a deep mark on the human heart. True courtesy asks us to pause. It teaches us that healing begins not with medicine, but with connection.

Respect should never depend on someone's background, condition, or education. A good doctor honours the dignity of every patient equally. Courteousness shows that we see them, not just the illness, but the person.

When someone is unwell, they are often scared and vulnerable. It is in these moments that our smallest acts become the most meaningful. Sitting beside them, not just treating the disease but holding space for their fears, their hopes—this is what sets a good doctor apart.

In truth, the best technologies and impressive hospital lobbies mean little if the patient feels unseen. Courteousness costs almost nothing but builds trust, encourages compliance, and lays the foundation for lasting doctor-patient rapport. Whether treating someone in an emergency room or a quiet clinic, let us not forget: a respectful gesture often heals before the medicine does.

CHAPTER 6

THE QUIET POWER OF PATIENCE

> Adopt the pace of nature: her secret is patience.
>
> – **Ralph Waldo Emerson**

In the fast pace of modern medicine, patience is not just a virtue. It is a necessity. Every patient who walks into your chamber is not just carrying symptoms; they carry fears and confusion. They have a story they want to tell. They don't just need a prescription. They need your time.

Often, we assume we have heard it all before. Chest pain, headaches, fatigue—it feels repetitive. But for the patient, it's new, it's worrying, and it matters deeply. If we rush them, interrupt them, or appear distracted, we diminish their sense of being heard. They begin to feel like a case, not a person.

Patience means allowing the patient to speak at their own pace, even when the story seems irrelevant or long, or repetitive. Sometimes, it is in those seemingly "unrelated" moments that they reveal the real clue. A missed word, an emotion behind a hesitation—it takes patience to catch it.

True healing begins when the patient feels that their doctor is not in a hurry. When they feel valued, they begin to trust. We all know trust is the foundation of every successful treatment.

Remember, your calm presence is more therapeutic than you know. Your ability to sit with their confusion without rushing, to repeat instructions without irritation, to listen without judgment—that's what patients remember long after the medicine is finished.

Patience is not about slowing down your day. It is about giving dignity to someone else's pain. Remember that sometimes, just being patient is the most powerful medicine you can give.

CHAPTER 7

TRUST: THE CORNERSTONE OF EFFECTIVE CLINICAL PRACTICE

> Trust is the glue of life. It's the most essential ingredient in effective communication. It is the foundational principle that holds all relationships.
>
> — **Stephen R. Covey**

Trust forms the backbone of the doctor–patient relationship. In a healthcare setting, patients find themselves vulnerable—physically, emotionally, and mentally. In such moments, trust is not just preferred; it is expected. Patients trust their healthcare providers to act in their best interests and deliver care that is competent, ethical, and dependable. This trust is not given lightly; it is earned through consistent actions, empathy, and professional conduct.

In medical literature, trust has been described in several ways. Some define it as a collection of expectations that a patient holds about their physician's behaviour. Others see it as a sense of reassurance or confidence that the doctor will deliver quality care. A more detailed perspective views trust as an unwritten agreement. It is an understanding that both the patient and the doctor will carry out their respective roles without fear of unexpected change. It is the patient's optimistic acceptance of vulnerability, believing that the doctor will act in their best interest, guided by goodwill and professional ethics.

To build this trust, doctors must listen actively. When a physician creates a safe space for open dialogue, patients feel free to discuss even the most personal and sensitive details. These conversations divulge critical informationthat significantly affects clinical decisions. If patients hold back, it may signal a gap in trust.

As a physician, the effort to earn and protect patient trust is continuous. Trust is not just a moral obligation; it is a clinical necessity. Building it takes time, but the benefits for both doctor and patient are lasting and profound.

CHAPTER 8

THE SILENT PROMISE: GUARDING WHAT PATIENTS TRUST US WITH

> Confidentiality is a virtue of the loyal, as loyalty is the virtue of faithfulness.
>
> **– Edwin Louis Cole**

Confidentiality is not just a legal obligation. It is a sacred bond. Every patient who sits before a doctor shares not just symptoms, but fears, histories, and vulnerabilities. This exchange is an act of profound trust, one that forms the core of the healing relationship.

One of the timeless principles of the Hippocratic Oath is confidentiality. It reminds us that what is heard in the sacred space between doctor and patient must never leave it. This is not merely about privacy laws. It is about dignity, respect, and empathy. In an age of electronic records and digital communication, protecting personal information has never been more challenging or more critical.

Doctors are often the last safe place in a patient's world. Breaching that trust, even unintentionally, can shatter more than confidence. It can hinder healing.

Let us remember: patients do not only trust us with their bodies. They entrust us with their stories, and by maintaining confidentiality, we preserve the soul of our profession.

Confidentiality is not just a rule. It is our quiet promise. A promise we must never break.

CHAPTER 9

EVEN A DISCOUNT CAN BE A BLESSING

> A small act of kindness can echo in a thousand hearts.

As doctors, we often meet patients who are not just physically unwell but also emotionally and financially burdened. A large number of people still live without any form of health insurance. Many more have government health cards that are not accepted at most private clinics. These patients often come to us with hesitation. Their eyes show a mix of hope for care and relief, and fear about whether they can afford the treatment. In that moment, they are not just looking for a doctor. They are looking for understanding and help.

Offering a discount or waiving certain fees for such patients is not about losing income. It is an act of service, grounded in humanity. When we ease their burden, even in small ways, we build trust that goes beyond any treatment. We become more than just healthcare providers. We become someone they can rely on.

These patients remember your kindness. They talk about it to their families, friends, and neighbours. Their blessings, genuine gratitude, and word-of-mouth referrals bring more people to your door than any paid advertisement ever could. This is how reputations are built-not through degrees on the wall, but through compassion in the heart.

Compassion is not a weakness. It doesn't lower the value of your service. In fact, it strengthens the foundation of your practice. When you care deeply and act kindly, you don't just heal bodies. You uplift lives. In return, your clinic becomes a place that truly serves the community, in every sense of the word.

CHAPTER 10

WHEN WORDS BECOME CARE: THE TRUE POWER OF DOCTOR-PATIENT DIALOGUE

> Words are, of course, the most powerful drug used by mankind.

– Rudyard Kipling

In the world of medicine, your words are as powerful as your prescriptions. Patients come to you not just seeking a cure, but also clarity, comfort, and compassion. Illness can suffocate even the bravest of souls, and your clinic may feel intimidating to someone anxious, afraid, or in pain.

Effective communication is one of the most important expectations patients have when they meet you. They look to you to explain their condition, guide them through treatment choices, and help them understand what lies ahead. A diagnosis may be complex, but your explanation shouldn't be. The last thing a patient should feel is confused when they leave your office.

Never hesitate to pause, rephrase, or repeat. A calm tone and empathetic approach can ease fears and build lasting trust. When patients feel heard and informed, they are more likely to follow treatment plans and achieve better outcomes.

Communication in healthcare is not an add-on—it is the foundation of good treatment. Your words can empower, comfort, and heal. Speak with empathy, and you will not only treat the illness but also care for the person behind it.

CHAPTER 11

TRUST BEGINS WITH TRUTH – THE ROLE OF TRANSPARENCY IN MEDICINE

> To be trusted is a greater compliment than to be loved.
>
> — **George MacDonald**

In every doctor-patient relationship, honesty forms the strongest bridge. Neither do patientsexpect their doctors to know everything, nor do they believe that doctors are free from error. What they truly value is transparency. A clear, honest conversation about their health, their disease, and the road ahead.

When a diagnosis remains uncertain, it is better to say so than to hide behind vague language. As doctors, we must communicate what we do know and acknowledge what we don't. Patients understand that uncertainty is part of life and medicine. Uncertainty is acceptable as long as we speak the truth.

A patient feels reassured when the doctor explains the nature of the disease in simple, clear terms. They appreciate learning about the treatment options, success rates, and possible risks. When they receive full information, they feel included in their own care.

Patients also know that doctors are human. They do not expect perfection. Most patients do not seek punishment when an error occurs. But they do expect their doctor to own up to it. When we admit a mistake and show our effort to fix it, we regain their trust.

Transparency builds confidence and strengthens rapport. It turns difficult conversations into meaningful connections. A well-informed patient is not only calmer but also more cooperative. Honesty does not weaken a doctor's image. It improves it.

In our practice, let us remember: truth heals. When we speak clearly, admit our limits, and guide with openness, we do more than treat illness. We build trust, and trust in medicine is the first step towards healing.

CHAPTER 12

EMERGENCY SERVICES-
WHEN EVERY SECOND COUNTS

> In an emergency, the first five minutes can write the story of a lifetime.

– Anonymous.

*I*n the life of a doctor, some moments call not just for skill, but for swiftness — for stepping out of routine, and responding to the cry of urgency.

In emergencies, time is life. Patients and their families do not look at your clock. They look at you with hope. A delay, even of seconds, can change the course of a life. What seems like a simple arm or chest pain might be a heart attack waiting to strike hard. Your timely presence could be the shield that stops it.

Yes, routine OPDs and paperwork are important. But a doctor's greatest duty is to respond when life is on the edge. Ignoring such calls can lead not only to tragic outcomes but also to mistrust, anger, and irreversible damage to your reputation and practice.

Responding swiftly in emergencies is not just a medical responsibility. It is human compassion. It is a silent promise we make every day: when someone is in pain, we will be there — now, not later.

Emergencies do not wait for appointments. They come unannounced, demanding your full attention, your compassion, and above all, your speed.

Let your name be remembered not just as a healer, but as someone who never turned away.

CHAPTER 13

EMBRACING COLLABORATIVE CARE: THE ART OF TIMELY SECOND OPINIONS

> A timely second opinion turns doubt into confidence.
>
> **– Anonymous**

In the journey of medical practice, maintaining patient trust is paramount. Studies on patient expectations reveal that one of the clearest wishes patients express is for their physician to recognize when a fresh perspective is needed. When faced with a challenging case, the most compassionate act is to seek a colleague's expertise without hesitation. Delaying a second opinion can not only prolong suffering but may also erode the hard-won confidence a patient has placed in you.

Once their condition improves, these patients frequently return, grateful for your honesty and commitment to their well-being. By demonstrating openness to collaboration, you strengthen the therapeutic alliance and underscore the shared goal of optimal care.

Remember: medicine is not a solitary endeavour. It thrives on the collective wisdom of our community. When a case exceeds our expertise, swift consultation can mean the difference between prolonged illness and timely recovery. Encourage dialogue, respect your colleagues' insights, and foster an environment where seeking help is seen not as weakness, but as the hallmark of a truly devoted physician.

CHAPTER 14

THE TRUE MEASURE OF CARE – BEING THERE WHEN IT MATTERS MOST

> A healing hand delayed is a healing hope lost. Be there, always.

In the journey of healing, one of the greatest gifts a doctor can offer a patient is simple yet profound, and that is availability.

Studies on patient expectations consistently reveal that one of the biggest causes of dissatisfaction is not the quality of treatment, but the difficulty in reaching the doctor when they are most needed. Long waiting times, delayed appointments, and inaccessibility during critical moments leave patients feeling abandoned and vulnerable.

If a patient is ill and needs your care, your presence should not depend on the hour of the day or your personal schedule. Whether it is lunchtime, your gym hour, or late evening, if a patient needs you, you must be there.

For what use is a doctor who is absent when healing hands are most needed?

Easy access to appointments and quick responses to concerns greatly enhance patient satisfaction. It deepens trust and strengthens the doctor-patient bond. On the other hand, long wait times, delayed responses, and limited availability often lead to frustration. It leads to eroded trust and patients seeking help elsewhere.

Yes, improving your availability may add to your workload, pressure, and even stress. But it also lays the foundation for a practice built on genuine trust, gratitude. All this can lead to lasting success.It is not the luxurious clinic or the latest technology that stays in a patient's memory — it is your presence at their hour of need.

In the end, being available is not just a professional duty; it is a sacred promise — to stand by those who entrust you with their health, their fears, and their hopes.

CHAPTER 15

SETTING UP NEXT APPOINTMENTS-BEYOND THE FIRST VISIT

> Without continuity, care loses its meaning.

A patient's journey doesn't end when they leave your consultation room. In fact, that's just one part of their healing process. As doctors, we carry the responsibility to guide them through every step of their care,even after the visit is over. One important and often overlooked step is scheduling the next appointment before they walk out.

This small gesture creates a sense of continuity and builds trust. It shows that we care about their progress and are committed to seeing them through their recovery. When a follow-up is clearly planned, patients are more likely to stay involved in their treatment and less likely to forget or delay care.

Without a proper follow-up plan, many patients drop out of treatment too early. Their symptoms may return, worsen, or go unnoticed. Timely follow-ups help us check their progress, make needed changes, and catch early signs of problems. It is not just about keeping our schedules full. It is about keeping our patients well.

Taking this extra step shows professionalism, care, and responsibility. In the long run, it leads to better health outcomes and stronger doctor-patient relationships. A scheduled follow-up is a promise and a quiet reminder that their health still matters to you.

CHAPTER 16

DISEASE FOLLOW-UP: THE SILENT STRENGTH OF GOOD MEDICINE

> Recovery begins with treatment but lasts through follow-up.

A diagnosis is not the end. It is the beginning of a responsibility. A physician must not only identify disease but also monitor its course with diligence and empathy. Regular follow-up bridges the gap between treatment and recovery. It ensures timely intervention, builds trust, and improves outcomes. Patients feel seen, not just checked. Chronic or acute, each condition evolves, and so must our attention to it. True care lies in consistency. Follow-up is not optional. It is integral to healing.

Follow-up care ensures that treatment is working, side effects are managed, and the patient's condition is truly understood. It offers timely opportunities to adjust medications, revisit lifestyle changes, and provide emotional reassurance.

Patients feel truly cared for when their doctor remembers, checks in, and listens. They feel seen, not just as cases, but as individuals. This builds conviction, which is as powerful as the medicine itself.

Consistency is the heart of good healthcare. A single consultation cannot replace the value of continued care. Follow-up is not optional—it is a vital part of the healing process. It reflects a physician's true dedication to health, comfort, and long-term recovery. Through every follow-up, we show that we are not just treating, but truly caring.

SECTION 2

A GOOD DOCTOR'S QUALITY

CHAPTER 1

PHYSICIAN COMPETENCY - THE ART OF EXPERTISE IN TREATMENT

> Medicine is not only a science; it is also an art. It does not consist of compounding pills and plasters; it deals with the very processes of life.
>
> **– Paracelsus**

Competence is not a mere expectation in medicine. It is the foundation. As the first and most vital pillar of a physician's professional identity, clinical expertise defines how trust is earned, how lives are improved, and how the dignity of care is upheld.

The modern physician must possess more than theoretical knowledge. They must actively apply it with precision, empathy, and adaptability.

To be truly expert at treatment, a physician must combine up-to-date medical knowledge with sound clinical judgment. Mastery in diagnostics, choice of therapies, and timing of interventions are not optional. They are essential. Treatment begins not with a prescription but with a deep understanding of the patient's unique condition, context, and concerns. This level of care demands ongoing learning, skill refinement, and emotional intelligence.

Physician competency also means recognising the limits of one's expertise and knowing when to consult or refer. It includes effective communication with patients and families, ensuring that every treatment plan is not only medically sound but clearly understood and respected.

Excellence in treatment does not happen by chance. It is a discipline, a responsibility, and above all, a commitment—to the science of healing and the art of caring.

CHAPTER 2

CHAPTER TITLE: COMPASSION – A DOCTOR'S MOST POWERFUL SKILL

> They may forget your name, but they will never forget how you made them feel.
>
> – **Maya Angelou**

We have already spoken about compassion in the earlier section on patient expectations. But some qualities are so important that they deserve to be repeated. Compassion is one of them. Without it, no doctor can truly connect with their patient. That is why we are touching on this aspect again. This is because no list of essential doctor qualities can be complete without it.

Compassion allows a doctor to see the person beyond the illness. It is the quiet understanding, the gentle tone, the extra moment spent explaining, and the willingness to listen without rushing. Patients often come with pain, fear, or confusion. Compassion is what makes them feel heard, comforted, and safe.

When doctors show compassion, they do more than treat disease—they heal people. It improves trust, builds better relationships, and helps patients follow treatment plans more willingly. It also reminds doctors why they chose this path: to help, to care, and to serve with kindness. In busy hospital corridors and demanding clinics, compassion might feel like a luxury. But in truth, it is a necessity. It is not a weakness. It is a strength, and the mark of a truly good doctor.

CHAPTER 3

HEALING WITH RESPECT: UNDERSTANDING DIVERSITY IN MEDICAL PRACTICE

> It is not our differences that divide us. It is our inability to recognize, accept, and celebrate those differences.
>
> **– Audre Lorde**

A truly effective doctor does more than diagnose and prescribe. A great doctor recognises the unique identity of each patient, acknowledging their age, gender, religion, and cultural background. These elements shape a patient's understanding of illness, health beliefs, and trust in treatment.

Respecting elderly patients means taking extra time, speaking clearly, and listening patiently. With children, it calls for gentleness, reassurance, and involving the parents. Gender sensitivity can influence communication and comfort, especially during examinations or discussions about reproductive health.

Religion may affect decisions on procedures, medication, or even the timing of care. Understanding and accommodating such beliefs, where possible, shows respect and builds trust. Culture also influences diet, lifestyle, and attitudes towards medical intervention.

When doctors approach every patient without judgment and with open-minded care, they don't just treat bodies, they honour lives. In today's diverse society, culturally competent care is not just ethical. It is essential.

By accepting differences and showing empathy, doctors create an environment where every patient feels seen, safe, and respected. This, in turn, improves cooperation, healing, and the human connection at the heart of medicine.

CHAPTER 4

FRIENDLY CHARISMA IN THE WHITE COAT

> A warm smile is the universal language of kindness.
>
> – **William Arthur Ward**

In every consultation room, there is more than just a doctor and a patient. There is a human connection waiting to be made. Friendly charisma is not about being overly familiar. It is about showing sincere warmth, patience, and presence. A kind greeting, a soft tone, and an open posture can instantly ease a patient's fear.

When doctors treat each patient with friendliness, they do more than deliver care. They create trust. That trust leads to open dialogue, better understanding of symptoms, and stronger compliance with treatment plans. Friendly behavior does not delay work. It makes it smoother and effective.

A doctor who listens with genuine interest and responds with empathy builds a relationship that goes beyond clinical duty. Even in the busiest hospitals, small acts of friendliness make a big difference. Patients remember how they felt more than what they heard.

Kindness is not a skill. It is a strength. It turns a routine visit into a meaningful exchange and makes healing feel personal. In a world where technology advances every day, the charm of human kindness remains irreplaceable.

CHAPTER 5

COURTEOUSNESS: THE QUIET STRENGTH OF A GREAT HEALER

> Kind words can be short and easy to speak, but their echoes are truly endless.
>
> **– Mother Teresa**

Courteousness may seem like a soft skill, but for a doctor, it holds great power. Patients remember how a doctor made them feel, more than what was said. While we have seen earlier how patients value respectful behavior, it is equally vital to understand why this trait is essential for the physician.

A courteous doctor builds trust faster. Clear, respectful communication opens doors to better compliance, smoother teamwork, and fewer conflicts. When doctors treat colleagues, patients, and support staff with courtesy, they create a safer environment where healing begins with connection.

Even in high-stress moments, a courteous approach shows control, maturity, and empathy. It makes difficult conversations easy and without any damage. Courteousness isn't weakness; it is a sign of a refined professional. It earns lasting respect not just from patients, but from peers and juniors too.

CHAPTER 6

EMBRACING CULTURAL SENSITIVITY IN HEALTHCARE

> A nation's culture resides in the hearts and the soul of its people.
>
> – **Mahatma Gandhi.**

In today's healthcare settings, cultural sensitivity is no longer optional; itis essential. As patient populations grow increasingly diverse, physicians must develop a deep understanding of cultural backgrounds, beliefs, and practices. A culturally sensitive doctor listens without judgment, respects patients' values, and adapts care plans to fit individual needs.

Effective communication forms the foundation of culturally competent care. Patients from different backgrounds may have varied expectations around treatment, consent, or family involvement. Doctors must remain open, ask the right questions, and avoid assumptions. Respecting a patient's culture strengthens trust, improves compliance, and leads to better outcomes.

Cultural awareness is equally important within the healthcare team. Physicians work alongside nurses, specialists, and support staff from different regions and cultures. Understanding and appreciating diverse communication and work styles fosters better teamwork and collaboration.

Doctors who embrace cultural inclusiveness not only enhance the patient experience but also help build a supportive and respectful clinical environment. By recognizing and valuing diversity in patients and colleagues, physicians can offer truly personalised care and contribute to a healthier, more united workplace.

CHAPTER 7

LAUGHTER IN THE WHITE COAT: LIGHTER SIDE OF CARE

> A good laugh heals a lot of hurts.
>
> **– Madeleine L'Engle**

*I*n the demanding world of medicine, a sense of humour can act as a shield and a bridge. For doctors, humour brings lightness to difficult situations and nurtures stronger connections with patients, families, and healthcare teams. When used with care, it humanises the doctor's role, builds trust, and encourages openness from those in their care. It also supports mental well-being and reduces burnout.

To develop this skill, doctors can start by observing humor in daily situations, reflecting on patient interactions, and engaging in team conversations with warmth. Sharing appropriate light-hearted moments can break tension and bring teams closer. In multidisciplinary teams, humour helps ease communication barriers, promotes collaboration, and builds resilience during tough times.

By using humor as a social tool, not just a personal trait, doctors can create more connected, compassionate, and collaborative care environments.

CHAPTER 8

INTEGRITY AND PROFESSIONALISM: THE PILLARS OF MEDICAL PRACTICE

> Real integrity is doing the right thing, knowing that nobody's going to know whether you did it or not.
>
> **– Oprah Winfrey**

*I*n medicine, integrity is more than a virtue. It is a professional obligation. Patients entrust their lives to physicians, expecting honesty and a commitment to their well-being. Every clinical decision, every note written, and every conversation held reflects a physician's values. Professionalism, meanwhile, acts as the visible arm of integrity. It is seen in punctuality and respectful communication. It is also seen in maintaining patient confidentiality and adhering to evidence-based care.

Physicians face complex choices, where the right path is not always the easiest. In those moments, integrity demands transparency and courage. Upholding high ethical standards, especially when no one is watching, builds deep-rooted trust. It reassures patients that their doctor places their best interests above all else. Doctors can show their integrity by being honest with patients, even when delivering difficult news. They can also demonstrate it by making clinical decisions based on evidence, not convenience or pressure.

Among peers, professionalism earns respect and encourages a culture of accountability.

The principles of integrity and professionalism are not just about conduct; they are about character. In every consultation and decision, they remind us why we chose this noble profession.

CHAPTER 9

SHARPENING THE MIND: CRITICAL THINKING AND PROBLEM-SOLVING IN PRACTICE

> It is not enough to do your best; you must know what to do, and then do your best.
>
> **– W. Edwards Deming**

In the life of a doctor, critical thinking is more than a skill. It is a daily necessity. Each patient presents a unique puzzle, often with multiple possibilities and no clear answers. Good doctors approach these situations by asking the right questions, weighing evidence carefully, and not jumping to conclusions. They practice looking beyond the obvious and consider how symptoms connect in complex ways.

Problem-solving flows naturally from critical thinking. It demands creativity, flexibility, and clinical judgment. Doctors improve this skill by reflecting on past cases, learning from peers, and staying updated with medical advances. On-the-job challenges offer real-life opportunities to fine-tune decisions.

Doctors should practise slowing down during routine cases, analysing why they chose one path over another. Even small actions like choosing when to refer or when to wait can shape patient outcomes. A great doctor recognises that each choice carries weight and continuously works to improve how they make those choices.

Over time, critical thinking becomes second nature, and problem-solving turns into a reliable tool. But this only happens when doctors treat every case, no matter how simple, as a chance to think better and act wiser.

CHAPTER 10

GROWING WITH GRACE – THE LIFELONG JOURNEY OF A HEALER

> A good doctor is not the one who knows everything, but the one who never stops learning.

In the world of medicine, the only constant is change. New research, fresh protocols, and changing technologies keep shifting the ground beneath our feet. But a doctor's true strength lies in their ability to grow, adapt, and rise with these changes. Lifelong learning is not just about attending conferences or reading journals. It is a mindset. It is the quiet promise we make to our patientsthat we will never stop improving for them.

Adaptability is equally essential. A doctor who stays open, flexible, and curious can navigate unexpected challenges with grace. From fresh graduates to seasoned experts, every stage of a medical career demands humility and the courage to learn.

To build this skill, doctors can commit to small daily learning habits like reading one article a day, discussing cases with colleagues, or learning from mistakes without ego. Embracing feedback and stepping outside comfort zones helps, too. Medicine may change, but the doctor who keeps evolving always stays relevant, trusted, and deeply human.

In choosing lifelong learning, we honour both our science and our oath—to always do better, for those who count on us the most.

CHAPTER 11

EMBRACING INNOVATION: THE PULSE OF PROGRESS

> Innovation distinguishes between a leader and a follower.
>
> **– Steve Jobs**

In medicine, standing still is not an option. The most impactful doctors do more than heal — they innovate. Whether it's exploring new treatments, embracing advanced technologies, or adapting faster methods for better care, their curiosity shapes the future of healthcare. Dedication to innovation means choosing growth over comfort, learning over routine, and purpose over fear. It is this mindset that sets exceptional doctors apart. They don't just follow medical breakthroughs; they create them. In doing so, they make sure that their patients receive care that's not only current but truly cutting-edge. For a physician, innovation is not a luxury; it is a responsibility. Those who embrace it stay ahead, lead with purpose, and leave a legacy of progress in the lives they touch.

This drive to innovate does not always require grand inventions. Sometimes, it begins with small changes in daily practice — trying a new approach with a complex case, applying new research to improve outcomes, or finding ways to reduce patient wait times through better scheduling. Innovation often comes from asking, "Can this be done better?" and having the courage to test the answer.

In hospitals, clinics, and operating rooms, doctors who welcome change help improve systems that have stayed the same for years. They bring fresh thinking into areas where habits once ruled. Even in busy routines, they find moments to improve, question, and refine. This attitude creates a ripple effect. One small improvement can lead to better results for many. In this way, innovation becomes part of everyday care. It becomes a habit, not just an idea, and patients feel the benefit of that forward-thinking mindset every single day.

CHAPTER 12

THE ART OF PRECISION: MASTERING ATTENTION TO DETAIL

> Excellence is in the details. Give attention to the details, and excellence will come.
>
> **– Perry Paxton**

As doctors, we know that in our profession, every small detail holds immense value. A single missed symptom, a decimal in the wrong place, or a misread report can have life-altering consequences. That is why attention to detail is not just a skill — it is a duty. Physicians who stay meticulous and organised can diagnose more accurately, reduce medical errors, and offer truly high-quality care. It is not about perfectionism, but about being precise where it matters most. After all, doctors are trusted not just with treatment, but with lives. The ability to observe keenly, record correctly, and follow through thoroughly is what distinguishes a good doctor from a great one. In medicine, it is the little things that make the biggest difference.

In today's fast-paced medical environment, where patients present with complex histories and time is often limited, attention to detail becomes even more crucial. A thorough review of past-records, careful listening during consultations, and clear documentation can reveal patterns or risks that are not immediately obvious. It may be recognising a subtle change in a patient's condition or catching an inconsistency in lab results. These small observations can lead to quicker diagnoses and better outcomes. Moreover, clear and precise communication with colleagues, nurses, and patients reduces misunderstandings and provides continuity of care. Even in high-pressure settings like emergency departments or operating theatres, the ability to stay focused on details can prevent costly mistakes.

Ultimately, patients place their trust in doctors not just for their knowledge, but for their diligence. A commitment to detail shows care, builds confidence, and above all, saves lives — making it an essential pillar of medical professionalism.

CHAPTER 13

THE ART OF THOROUGH EXAMINATION

> Listen to your patient; they are telling you the diagnosis.
>
> **– Sir William Osler**

In clinical practice, a thorough examination is not just a routine step. It is the bedrock of accurate diagnosis and successful treatment. A good doctor begins by actively listening to the patient. Every detail matters—symptoms, duration, lifestyle, and family history all serve as valuable clues. This careful information gathering reflects the physician's intent to treat the whole patient, not just the illness.

After history taking, the physical examination follows. A skilled doctor uses clinical methods—observing the tongue, listening with the stethoscope, palpating areas of concern—to form a provisional diagnosis. This physical interaction helps build trust. The patient feels seen, heard, and respected.

Sometimes, initial clinical findings may not be conclusive. That is when investigations, such as blood tests or scans, come into play. However, without a solid foundation laid through proper examination and history-taking, even tests may mislead. It is often said that “what you miss in history, you won’t find in the lab.”

Even in cases where the diagnosis is elusive, a doctor must reflect: Was something overlooked in the examination? Thoroughness is not a habit; it is a discipline. It defines the doctor’s dedication to the truth hidden within each patient.

When a doctor listens, observes, and examines with care, the body reveals what words often hide. A missed step in examination can echo as a missed opportunity for healing.

CHAPTER 14

THE TRUE ROLE OF A DOCTOR: MORE THAN A PRESCRIPTION

> An ounce of prevention is worth a pound of cure.
>
> – **Benjamin Franklin**

A good doctor is not someone who just writes a prescription and sends the patient away. The real role of a doctor is much bigger. A doctor must think about the patient's lifestyle, habits, and daily routine. Many health problems today are caused by how we live—poor diet, no exercise, stress, or lack of sleep. These are called lifestyle disorders.

A thoughtful doctor always advice on how to improve one's life. This includes eating better, exercising regularly, quitting smoking, and sleeping on time. Doctors are trained in social and preventive medicine so they can guide people to avoid getting sick in the first place. For example, when someone comes with malaria or dengue, it is not enough to just give medicine. A responsible doctor also explains how to stop mosquitoes from breeding and protect oneself with nets and repellents.

In conditions like diabetes, lifestyle changes such as better food choices and regular walking often help more than high doses of medicine. A wise doctor will first suggest these changes and add medicine only if needed. This helps keep the disease in control without harming the body with unnecessary drugs.

The goal of every doctor should be to help people stay healthy—not just treat them when they fall sick. Preventive care, lifestyle advice, and health education are just as important as writing the right prescription. A true doctor heals not just with medicines, but also with knowledge and guidance.

CHAPTER 15

WORDS THAT HEAL: MASTERING COMMUNICATION IN MEDICINE

> The single biggest problem in communication is the illusion that it has taken place.
>
> **– George Bernard Shaw**

Clear and compassionate communication is a core part of being a good doctor. It is not enough to have all knowledge. One must also know how to share it. When a doctor simply explains complex medical terms, patients feel understood and safe. Strong communication helps avoid confusion, reduces fear, and builds trust. It also strengthens teamwork among healthcare professionals, leading to better care.

Doctors can improve communication by actively listening to patients, watching their body language, and giving them time to speak. Speaking slowly, using common words, and checking if the patient has understood the message is key. Communication training should not stop after medical school. Doctors must continue to reflect on how they speak and how they are heard.

Practising empathy and staying calm, even in stressful situations, can greatly improve doctor–patient relationships.

In every patient meeting, a doctor must not only diagnose but also connect. Words, when used with care, can heal alongside medicine.

CHAPTER 16

IN THEIR CORNER: A COMMITMENT TO ADVOCACY IN MEDICINE

> The best interest of the patient is the only interest to be considered.
>
> **– William Mayo**

True commitment to patient advocacy means always placing the patient's well-being at the centre of care. In today's complex healthcare systems, it's not enough to diagnose and treat; physicians must also guide, support, and protect patients,especially those who are vulnerableand uninformed. Advocacy involves helping patients understand their treatment options, speaking up for their rights, and ensuring they receive the care they deserve, even in difficult or bureaucratic circumstances.

From the Hippocratic Oath to modern-day hospital ethics, patient advocacy remains a foundational pillar. It demands empathy, patience, and the courage to act in the patient's best interest—even when it requires challenging systems or decisions.

Doctors can develop this essential skill by actively listening to patients, staying informed about health policies and resources, and building strong, trust-based relationships. Regular reflection on patient interactions and engaging in ethics training also strengthens this commitment. Above all, advocacy must become a mindset where every decision and conversation is shaped by the question: "What is best for my patient?"

CHAPTER 17

STANDING STRONG AGAINST PRESSURE FROM PHARMACEUTICAL COMPANIES

> The first wealth is health.
>
> **– Ralph Waldo Emerson**

A doctor's first duty is to the patient—not to profit and not to pharma, but to healing. In today's world, pharmaceutical companies try hard to influence medical practice. They offer gifts, trips, and sponsorships to win favour, but a doctor must stand firm. Prescribing should always be based on the patient's best interest, not on pressure from marketing representatives.

Some physicians allow only top pharmaceutical brands, fearing generics may lead to bad results. While quality matters deeply, the key is to assess the medicine itself—not the company logo behind it. There are cases where specialists lost their practice because they prescribed low-quality drugs under the influence of companies. This is a mistake we must learn from.

Doctors should never compromise on quality or be swayed by pharma offers. The role of medical representatives is to inform—not to dictate. Even when a cheaper medicine works better, it is rarely promoted, because companies care more about profits than people.

True independence lies in making decisions based on science, ethics, and patient welfare. A doctor should never forget that they work for humanity. Medicine must be a mission—not a market. Let health always come before wealth.

CHAPTER 18

LEADING WITH PURPOSE IN MEDICINE

> Leadership is not about being in charge. It is about taking care of those in your charge.
>
> – **Simon Sinek**

In healthcare, leadership goes beyond titles or authority. It is about responsibility, vision, and empathy. Doctors often find themselves leading teams, guiding junior colleagues, or setting the tone during high-pressure situations. Strong leadership helps build a culture of trust, respect, and teamwork. It inspires teams to work with purpose and align around patient-centred goals.

Doctors can develop leadership skills by practising active listening, encouraging open dialogue, and giving constructive feedback. Leading by example—through professionalism, accountability, and kindness—promotes unity in healthcare settings. Attending leadership workshops, seeking mentorship, and reflecting on both successes and failures can further strengthen this quality.

A doctor-leader lifts others, ensures every voice is heard, and maintains calm in crisis. When doctors lead well, teamwork improves, staff morale rises, and patient care becomes safer and more effective. True leadership in medicine lies not in control but in building others up for the greater good.

CHAPTER 19

MASTERING TIME: THE KEY TO BALANCE IN MEDICINE

> Time is what we want most, but what we use worst.
>
> **–William Penn**

*I*n the life of a doctor, every minute counts. Between patient consultations, clinical documentation, administrative work, and ongoing learning, physicians often feel pulled in many directions. Good time management helps doctors stay focused, reduce stress, and maintain the quality of care their patients deserve. When time is managed well, doctors can respond more effectively to urgent situations. They can make space for thoughtful, compassionate care.

Equally important is the need to protect personal well-being, without regular breaks and moments to reset, fatigue and burnout can quietly take hold. A short pause during a demanding shift can help improve focus, mood, and decision-making. Time set aside for self-care is not selfish. It is essential for sustainability in such a high-pressure profession.

To develop strong time management skills, doctors can start by identifying priorities, setting realistic goals, and creating structured routines. Using digital tools or checklists can also improve efficiency. Most importantly, building the habit of stepping back, even briefly, lets physicians return with greater clarity and calm. In the end, managing time wisely means giving the best to both patients and oneself.

CHAPTER 20

RESILIENCE AND EMOTIONAL STAMINA: THE HEART OF A HEALER

> It's not the load that breaks you down, it's the way you carry it.
>
> **– Lou Holtz**

In the life of a physician, every day brings emotional weight—whether it is breaking difficult news, managing critical cases, or enduring long, unpredictable hours. Resilience is the quiet strength that helps doctors remain composed amidst chaos, while emotional stamina sustains them through the relentless demands of their role.

Those who embrace humour and find moments of lightness in their work are more fulfilled. A shared laugh with a colleague or a moment of reflection can soften the edges of stress. Over time, these simple joys become powerful tools for self-preservation.

Doctors can nurture resilience and stamina by practising mindfulness, building strong peer support, getting adequate rest, and making room for hobbies. A balanced life beyond the clinic helps healers stay whole—because to care for others, they must also care for themselves.

SECTION 3

THE LITTLE THINGS THAT COUNT MOST

CHAPTER 1

THE WAITING ROOM WHISPER – CREATING TRUST FROM THE FRONT DESK

> Kindness is a language that the deaf can hear and the blind can see.
>
> **– Mark Twain**

The patient's journey doesn't begin in the consultation room. It starts the moment they enter the clinic. For many, the front desk is the first human contact they encounter. In this moment, a warm reception becomes more than just good manners. It becomes a key part of the healing process.

Medical environments can be intimidating. Patients arrive feeling unwell, anxious, or uncertain. A friendly smile, a gentle tone, and a welcoming attitude from reception staff can immediately ease stress. These small acts of kindness create a sense of comfort and belonging. This can directly influence how patients perceive the entire practice.

These days, patients are twice as likely to choose or avoid a doctor based on the friendliness and professionalism of the front-desk team. This means the role of the receptionist is no longer solely administrative; it is also relational. How patients are welcomed can shape their overall trust in the care they are about to receive.

Doctors must lead the way by setting expectations for a respectful and empathetic reception culture. Front desk staff should be trained not just in systems and scheduling. But also in emotional intelligence and patient interaction. A positive first impression can calm nerves, reduce fear, and help patients feel seen and heard before a single medical word is spoken.

The emotional atmosphere of the reception area reflects directly on the doctor's professionalism and care.This shift highlights the fact that clinical excellence alone is no longer enough. Patients expect empathy from the entire care team.

In short, the welcome at the door can echo all the way into recovery.

CHAPTER 2

STAFFING CHOICES THAT SHAPE OR SHATTER A DOCTOR'S LEGACY

> It takes 20 years to build a reputation and five minutes to ruin it.
>
> **– Warren Buffett**

*I*n the medical world, where every decision can impact a life, the value of a well-qualified, and experienced team cannot be overstated. While infrastructure and technology matter, it is the people—your staff—who carry your vision into practice. Hiring unqualified or undertrained personnel for the sake of cutting costs may seem like a short-term solution, but it often becomes an expensive mistake.

Unqualified staff can compromise patient safety through poor handling, incorrect procedures, or missed signs. One of the most overlooked consequences is the increased risk of cross-infection due to improper sterilization techniques—something no clinic or hospital can afford. Patients often come from varied settings, and this includes healthcare. When word spreads about poor hygiene or careless handling in your clinic, your reputation takes the hit, not theirs.

Doctors unknowingly suffer the consequences of poor staffing. Patients lose trust. Referrals stop. Your professional image, carefully built over the years, may get tarnished by someone else's incompetence.

Especially in indoor hospital settings, where round-the-clock care is critical, unqualified staff become liabilities. A minor error can quickly escalate into a crisis. Sadly, it's the doctor, who is held accountable.

On the other hand, experienced and qualified staff may come at a higher cost, but they elevate your practice. Their training, clinical acumen, and ability to handle high-pressure situations not only ensure patient safety but also enhance the overall standard of care. Ultimately, they protect your image, support your decisions, and uphold the dignity of your profession.

Choose your team wisely, because your name is only as strong as those who represent it.

CHAPTER 3

CLEANLINESS IS CARE: THE DOCTOR'S SILENT PROMISE

> Cleanliness is the hallmark of perfect standards, and the best quality inspector is the conscience.
>
> **– J.R.D. Tata**

A clean and well-kept clinic is more than just a reflection of hygiene. It is a reflection of a doctor's commitment to quality and patient care. In the healthcare sector, cleanliness is not a secondary concern; it is central to the patient experience, the reputation of the doctor, and the prevention of infections.

When a patient walks into a clinic, the first thing they notice is the environment. A tidy reception area, clean floors, fresh air, and organised spaces instantly convey professionalism and care. On the other hand, unclean clinics with stained walls, overflowing dustbins, or worse—red spit stains from chewing tobacco or betel leaf—can repel patients. Some may even walk away without meeting the doctor, simply due to poor aesthetics and hygiene.

Beyond perception, cleanliness has a direct impact on health outcomes. Hospital-acquired infections are a real threat. Maintaining sterile conditions and routine sanitisation can significantly reduce these risks. A good doctor understands that healing begins the moment a patient steps inside the facility.

Cleanliness must extend to every corner: sanitized instruments, clean examination beds, hand hygiene, proper waste disposal, and regular deep cleaning of high-touch surfaces. Staff should also follow hygiene protocols and wear clean uniforms.

Ultimately, cleanliness is not just the job of support staff. It is a standard that the doctor must set and uphold. A clean clinic is a silent but powerful way of saying, "Here, your health matters."

CHAPTER 4

CLEAN MEANS CREDIBLE: THE FIRST RULE OF MEDICAL PRACTICE

> Hygiene is two-thirds of health, a Lebanese proverb.

The moment a patient walks into a clinic, they begin to observe. A doctor's appearance—neatly groomed hair, clean clothes, polished shoes—speaks louder than any prescription. If a physician appears unhygienic or careless, trust begins to fade, even before the consultation begins.

In the field of medicine, personal hygiene is not just about self-care is a message. It is the foundation of social and preventive medicine taught early in medical education. A doctor must practice the same hygiene they advise their patients to follow. Daily bathing, handwashing, oral hygiene, trimmed nails, and clean clothing are not formalities; they are responsibilities.

Coughing and sneezing etiquette, sanitising equipment, and keeping the clinical environment clean protect the healer and the healed. Proper waste disposal, covered bins, and cleanliness in patient areas are critical. Waste management is not separate from personal hygiene—it is an extension of it.

A good doctor sets the standard. Excellence is not just in knowledge, but in habits. Cleanliness reflects discipline, care, and respect for human life. It builds trust and reassures the patient that they are in safe, capable hands. A clean doctor is a credible doctor.

CHAPTER 5

TOOLS THAT BUILD TRUST – THE VALUE OF GOOD MEDICAL EQUIPMENT

> A craftsman is only as good as his tools.

In today's world, patients not only seek expert care but also expect a clinic that reflects precision, trust, and advancement. One of the first things a patient notices is your equipment. A simple digital blood pressure monitor attached to a multiparameter monitor often speaks louder than words. It tells the patient: "You are in safe, modern hands."

While conventional tools have served medicine for decades, modern devices add a sense of credibility in the eyes of patients. A well-functioning ECG machine, a clean pulse oximeter, or even a digital stethoscope creates a strong impression. It reassures the patient that their doctor values accuracy and stays updated with technology.

Of course, high-quality diagnostic equipment comes at a price. But it is not about comparison—it is about perception. When patients see digital tools, they believe their doctor is serious about both diagnosis and care. It enhances trust even before treatment begins.

Different specialties need different sets of equipment. A dermatologist, an ENT, a cardiologist, or a gynaecologist cannot function with the same tools. However, whatever the specialty, equipment must always be clean, sterilised, and ready to use. Sterility speaks of professionalism. Broken, outdated, or rusty equipment may send the wrong message.

Ultimately, patients may not understand the inner workings of a device, but they do understand what it represents: care, commitment, and class. Investing in quality medical equipment is not a luxury. It is a quiet promise of excellence.

CHAPTER 6

THE LIGHT THAT BUILDS TRUST – THE POWER OF THE MEDICAL PEN TORCH

> Excellence is in the details. Give attention to the details, and excellence will come.
>
> **– Perry Paxton**

In clinical practice, even the smallest tools can carry great weight. The medical pen torch, often overlooked, holds a key role in everyday patient care. As emphasized in Kapoor's Guide for General Practitioners—a 12-volume reference for every general physician—this tool is more than a light source; it is a symbol of clinical commitment.

The writer of this book was a Professor of Medicine at Grant Medical College, Mumbai, and a highly respected and capable figure in the field. Drawing from years of rich experience, he wrote what I have personally seen in clinical practice—that in a crowded dispensary, the only truly useful instrument is a powerful torch. A stethoscope, while helpful, is not always necessary.

During ENT examinations or skin assessments, the use of a torch allows for accurate diagnosis. More importantly, it gives the patient the impression that the doctor is attentive, careful, and genuinely invested. When a practitioner skips close examination and prescribes from a distance, patients often feel ignored or unsatisfied.

Even if the diagnosis seems obvious, using a torch confirms the clinical finding and strengthens patient confidence. A brief check under good light tells the patient, "You matter. I have taken the time." In a world where healthcare is precious, the pen torch can silently speak volumes.

Doctors must remember—it is not just about knowing the diagnosis; it is about showing the care. The pen torch, when used well, lights up more than just the body—it lights up patient faith.

CHAPTER 7

THE HUMAN TOUCH IN CLINICAL SPACE

> Too often we underestimate the power of a touch, a smile, a kind word... or the smallest act of caring, all of which have the potential to turn a life around.
>
> **– Leo Buscaglia.**

A patient once called me asking for a referral to a specialist. I suggested someone I trusted, but he hesitated. When I asked why, he said, "That doctor examines from a distance. The specialist hardly comes close." His response left a lasting impression. It reminded me that while professionalism is crucial, so is being approachable. Patients don't just seek medical expertise. They look for human connection. When a doctor stands too far, it can create not only physical but also emotional distance. That space can quietly erode trust, limit communication, and make the patient feel unseen.

Proximity fosters a sense of connection and empathy. When a doctor examines a patient from nearby, it silently says, "I care, and I am here with you." It enhances both the emotional and diagnostic aspects of care.

Of course, in cases involving infectious diseases, safety protocols are vital—masks, gloves, sanitiser, even shields if needed. But protection should never come at the cost of compassion. Patients, even those who are contagious, deserve to feel seen, heard, and valued.

The healing process begins not just with medicine, but with presence. Let us not allow fear or formality to create a barrier between us and those we serve.

CHAPTER 8

BEYOND THE CLINIC—A DOCTOR'S DUTY IN PATIENT TRANSPORTATION

> They alone live who live for others. The rest are more dead than alive.
>
> **– Swami Vivekananda**

Patient care doesn't end at diagnosis or prescription. True healing begins with compassion, and sometimes, that means stepping beyond clinical boundaries—especially in moments when time is life.

Doctors may not physically drive ambulances or push stretchers, but their role in ensuring safe and timely transportation for patients is critical. Imagine a patient who walks in complaining of mild chest pain. A vigilant doctor might recognize signs of a heart attack—at that moment, writing a prescription is not enough. Arranging for immediate transport, even if it means using one's own vehicle, can save a life.

Such acts speak volumes about a doctor's commitment to patient-centered care. Whether it's mobilizing the staff to handle stretchers or ensuring someone accompanies the patient to a diagnostic test from the IPD, this attention shows depth of care.

Trained assistance, proper planning, and a humane approach reflect a doctor's ability to navigate beyond medicine. This doesn't just build trust—it earns lasting goodwill. Because patients never forget the doctor who stood by them when they couldn't stand alone.

CHAPTER 9

LEADERSHIP IN THE WHITE COAT – RESPECTING THE TEAM BEHIND THE DOCTOR

> The strength of the team is each individual member. The strength of each member is the team.
>
> **– Phil Jackson**

A doctor who treats his medical staff as mere subordinates commits a serious professional and ethical error. The salary paid is not a license for arrogance. It is a fair exchange for skill, time, and dedication. A wise physician understands that mutual respect forms the foundation of a successful medical team.

The most admired doctors are not those who issue commands. But those who lead through active engagement and shared responsibility with their team. When the staff feels genuinely respected, they respond with loyalty, enthusiasm, and a willingness to go the extra mile even during the most demanding times. A doctor who listens to the appeals of his staff, who nurtures their growth, and who trusts their abilities, creates an environment where excellence is not enforced but inspired.

It is equally essential to maintain professionalism and grace in interactions with the opposite sex. Every colleague, regardless of gender, deserves courtesy, dignity, and a safe working space. Subtle disrespect or unchecked behaviour can undermine not only morale but also the sanctity of the workplace.

A good doctor does not merely command cooperation. They inspire it. True leadership lies in lifting others, cultivating potential, and creating an atmosphere where every member of the team feels valued and empowered.

CHAPTER 10

UPHOLDING THE HONOUR OF THE PROFESSION: CAMARADERIE AMONG DOCTORS

> Do unto others as you would have them do unto you.

The relationship between doctors must be built on mutual respect, loyalty, and discretion. While differences in opinion and approach are natural, criticism among colleagues must happen only in private and with complete confidence. To speak negatively about another doctor in front of a patient is not only damaging to the individual but also dangerous to the profession. It breaks trust, confuses the patient, and weakens the credibility of the medical community.

The Medical Council of India has declared in its Code of Medical Ethics:

"I will maintain by all means in my power, the honor and noble traditions of the medical profession."

It also affirms: "My colleagues will be my brothers." These aren't just lines to remember—they are promises we make to one another and society.

Similarly, the International Code of Ethics warns:

"A doctor must not entice patients away from his colleagues."

When a patient comes seeking a second opinion and speaks poorly of another doctor, listen with care—but never join in the criticism. At most, say that the doctor did what was right based on his or her assessment. If you cannot say anything kind, choose silence over disloyalty.

As doctors, our strength lies in standing together. A spirit of professional camaraderie not only honors our calling but ensures the best care for our patients.

CHAPTER 11

THE REFERRAL CIRCLE: BUILDING TRUST THROUGH RESPECTFUL COMMUNICATION

> Gratitude is not only the greatest of virtues, but the parent of all the others.
>
> – **Cicero**

When a doctor refers a patient, it is a gesture of trust. Acknowledging this trust is not just ethical, it is professional. One of the best ways to honour it is by expressing genuine gratitude to the patient and the referring doctor. A simple message or call, thanking the doctor for the referral, sets a respectful tone.

Communication must remain open. Keep the referring doctor informed—whether through a message, a WhatsApp update, or a phone call. If that's not possible, at least inform them when the patient visits and share relevant progress. This practice isn't just polite—it's smart. It strengthens professional ties and encourages more referrals in a competitive setting.

Avoid negative remarks about previous diagnoses or treatment. If there is a difference of opinion, present it with sensitivity. While speaking to the patient, always mention the role of the referring doctor. Show that their decision was correct and valued.

I know, a pediatrician regularly updates the referring doctor via phone or message—an example worth following. Acknowledgement, gratitude, and respectful updates are not just good habits; they form the foundation of a collaborative, respected medical practice.

CHAPTER 12

PROFESSIONAL COURTESY: A QUIET TRADITION OF RESPECT

> Courtesy among healers is not charity—it is character.

Extending professional courtesy to fellow doctors and their families is a long-standing and honourable tradition in medicine. Offering free consultations or discounted services not only reflects empathy and mutual respect. But also reinforces the values that bind the medical fraternity together.

Doctors who run private clinics or hospitals can consider offering free OPD services to other doctors and their immediate families. While IPD services may involve significant operational costs and cannot always be free, one can offer concessions on investigations, medicines, and final billing. This practice, rooted in ethics and goodwill, fosters a culture of trust, dignity, and unity.

Importantly, this should never be done with the sole expectation of future benefit. Rather, it must come from a place of sincere intention and moral responsibility. While such acts of kindness may bring goodwill or referrals down the line, the true value lies in nurturing the spirit of compassion within the profession.

In an increasingly commercialised environment, small sacrifices made for colleagues remind us of the nobility of our calling and that behind every white coat is a human heart that truly cares.